Anti-Aging
Homemade Remedies and Recipes
Age Gracefully, Look Younger and Live Longer

Disclaimer

The author has tried to be an authentic source of the information provided in this report. However, the author does not oppose the additional information available over the internet. The information included in this book cannot be compared with information of the same provided in other books. All readers can seek further help through additional sources of information.

Ignoring any of the guidelines for the tips or not following each step of the preparation method of the recipes may not give you the exact result. Therefore, the author is not responsible for such negligence.

Summary

Aging is indeed unavoidable and everyone faces it sooner or later. What really matters is to age gracefully and delay the dreadful signs of aging as much as possible. So whether it is the lines on your skin, the puffiness under the eyes, the unwanted wrinkles, graying hair or increasing pounds, you can control everything with the right approach.

In this book, we have covered everything you need to know about aging and the most effective anti-aging skin care, homemade remedies and super food recipes to help you age gracefully and beautifully.

In this book you will find:

1. The signs of aging and effective ways to avoid them
2. 10 interesting ways to defy your age naturally and enjoy more years of youthfulness
3. 40 tips to keep aging in your control
4. Homemade natural recipes from ingredients available in your kitchen for aging skincare
5. Skincare natural recipes from people around the world
6. Details on super foods, essential oil and herbs to help you look younger
7. Delicious and nutritionally rich anti-aging juicing recipes
8. Anti-aging food recipes to keep you fresh and young all these years

Ready to enjoy aging? Get started now!

Contents

Signs of Aging – The Best Way to Age Gracefully

A few lines here, a bag, or sag there – your body may be aging in not-so-graceful manner. While aging is an unavoidable situation one has to face in life, sometimes, the signs of aging can become so severe that it makes you look older than you actually are.

If this sounds like you, don't panic. Here we will discuss some of the best and most effective ways to fix these trouble spots. Read on!

Identifying and Fixing the Worse Signs of Aging

The following are some of the worse signs of aging that you must get rid of before it is too late.

1. Thinning, dull hair

Stress, certain medication, and childbirth are some factors that can cause hair loss as you age. In addition to this, hormonal shifts that you experience as a side effect of aging during menopause can also result in permanent hair thinning.

What to do?

First of all, test at home. Pull a small hank of hair beginning from the scalp to all the way to the tips of your hair. You have thinning problem if more than 6 hair come out. Check out for expert recommended products on the internet or see a doctor. Medicines and different organic oils can help you get rid of this problem so that you enjoy healthy, thick hair once again.

2. Turkey Neck

Aging can loosen your skin and can even lead to dreaded turkey neck. Aging can also make your skin very dry if you do not take proper care of it. Wrinkles and loosen skin can make you look older than your age.

What to do?

Pamper your skin and understand that it has become delicate with time. Use a nice moisturizer that is good for collagen production. As you treat your neck, keep it covered by wearing tops with ruffles or high-necks. Keeping a wrinkled neck covered can take 10 years of your age.

Some amazing, anti-aging moisturizer recipes are shared in this book to help you get rid of that turkey neck.

3. Spotted hands

Aging reduces the level of collagen in our body. This further leads to reduction in volume, making hands appear wrinkly with prominent veins. Sun damage marks and brown spots starts appearing too.

What to do?

Look for an effective sunscreen and apply on your hands daily, especially before going out in the sun. Keep your hands well moisturized to avoid dryness and wrinkles from appearing. Another great tip is to apply pale and nude nail polish shades to divert the focus from your hands. It looks more modern and classy.

4. Sore Feet

All your life, you stuffed your feet into extraordinary high heels and ill-fitting shoes. Time to repay all the punishment and treat your painful bunions, calluses, and cracked heels!

What to do?

Don't forget to take care of your feet and moisturize cracked heels before going to bed. Use comfortable shoes only. Look online to find brands offering comfortable, medicated shoes. Choosing shoes with Nike air cushion can greatly help you.

5. Wimpy lashes and brows

As you age, your hormone changes. This can even make your lashes and eyebrows sparse. Over tweezing your eyebrows all these years can affect the eyebrow follicles. Aging can make it difficult for the hair to grow back.

What to do?

You will use a cosmetic trick here to take off years from your face. Use an angled brush to fill the space between your eyebrows using a dark eye shadow color that matches with your hair.

As far as your lashes are concerned, use a good brand mascara to add volume to your eyes. You can even choose false lashes to make your lashes appear thick. Believe it or not, it can make a huge difference.

6. Winkled body

Wrinkles can travel from your face to all the way to your entire body. After all, who wants elephant knees or elbows? Aging skin creates wrinkles, and flaky, dry patches may easily appear.

What to do?

Pamper your dry skin with a good moisturizer (recipe shared below). Give yourself a nice, moisturizing body massage and relax yourself at the same moment.

7. Wrinkles and fine lines on the faces

Reduction in the level of elasticity and collagen can reduce the skin volume. This leads to wrinkles and fine lines. This could add a lot of age to your face.

What to do?

Prevention is the key here! Avoid squinting at the computer screen, or using straws to sip lattes or any repeated facial muscle movement that can stress the fine lines and wrinkles on your face. Also, make sure you have the skin-care basics with you, including moisturizer and sunscreen.

Defying Your Age Naturally: 8 Ways to Feel Younger without Pricey Treatments

While it is true that anti-aging procedures and cosmetics may play a significant role in slowing the process of again, there are a number of natural ways to do so. Natural ways allow you to feel younger, which is essential for looking younger as well.

Here's a rundown of the top 8 natural ways that allows you take a proactive approach to aging beautifully and gracefully.

Control How You Age: Adjusting Your Mindset

According to a research, serious aging occurs at cellular level. Our lifestyle habits, such as nutrition, sleep, stress management, and exercise are greatly responsible to enhance the ability of our body to repair the cellular damage that cannot be avoid as we age.

Thus, it is very important to adjust our mindset and identify the areas we need to work to slow down the process of aging and feel rejuvenated as we age. This mainly depends upon your lifestyle choices that will enhance the quality and length of your life.

Exercise Is Your Fountain of Youth

Begin with exercise! A good workout on a regular basis gives us a great sense of well-being. As natural age defyers, add the following exercises in your arsenal to keep you feeling and looking young.

1. Aerobic exercise
2. Strength Training
3. Daily Lifestyle Activities

Feed Your Face

Have you heard this common phrase, "you are what you eat?" This is absolutely true and you must focus on your nutrition as your anti-aging magic pill. There is a lot of information about the power of nutrition to enhance your well-being, boost your immune system, and to ward off illness.

Focus on your food and know what you are eating. Dirty junk food will not only add pounds to your body (making you look older), but will also affect your health and you may feel even older and weaker. Also, you need to maintain healthy skin in order to wipe of those bad wrinkles of your face naturally.

Food that is loaded with vitamins and polyphenois (anti-inflammatory properties and antioxidants that benefit and protect your skin) should be a part of your daily diet. The following is a list of delicious and colorful food that you can choose your daily nutrition from:

Vitamin A: Asparagus, bell peppers, carrot, cantaloupe, kale, spinach, leafy greens, broccoli, and sweet potatoes.

Vitamin C: Cantaloupe, oranges, kiwifruit, pineapple, strawberries, cauliflower, broccoli, and red bell pepper.

Vitamin E: Spinach, tomato products, vegetable oils, seeds and nuts.

Polypenols: dark chocolate, cocoa, and green tea.

Study and work on your balanced diet.

The Concept of Beauty Sleep

Stay up for several hours or experience a night of insomnia, and you will probably notice obvious signs of sleep deprivation on your face. Next morning, bags under the eyes and puffy eyes are a common sign that could make you feel ridiculous. Such signs are more than enough to make you feel tired and old.

Adjust your sleeping habit too to beautify yourself as you age. Make sure you get at least 7-8 hours of a good night sleep to rejuvenate yourself regardless of your age.

Deep Breathing, Yoga and Meditation

Use the calming method to take years away from your age. Unmanageable stress and age-related depression can wreak havoc on your body and make you feel older than you really are. It can even lead to high blood pressure, obesity, heart disease, and severe skin inflammation.

Anything you do to alleviate and manage stress will positively influence how you feel about yourself as you age. Yoga, meditation, and deep breathing exercise can be your solution. Dedicate a few minutes of each day to yourself. Stay quiet, center yourself, and let your stress drift away.

Make meditation and breathing exercises a part of your daily routine. Yoga will not only help you calm your mind, but will also keep your body strong and flexible – just like how you want to be in your old age.

Sun Protection for Your Skin

Nothing affects your aging skin faster than overexposure to the sun. In response to exposure of UV radiation, the level of collagen in our skin drops. It also affects the production of free radicals in our body, which further breaks down the level of collagen and damage cells in our body.

Avoid exposure to sun as much as possible. If it is unavoidable, make sure you put your sunscreen to good use.

Don't Forget Your Ears

When taking care of the skin, ears are the most neglected part of our face. There are very tiny hairs in our ears that respond to noise and we must clean and take care of our ears.

When moisturizing or applying any skincare treatment for aging, don't forget to apply some to your ears as well to have even and smooth skin throughout your face.

Limit Alcohol and Quit Smoking

Limit the consumption of alcohol as much as possible and try quitting smoking completely if you want to slow down the process of aging and improve your quality of life.

In addition to accelerating aging process, smoking can decrease lung capacity, cause heart disease and various other health conditions. Smoking is also associated with aging skin, yellowing of teeth, and wrinkles around the lips area. Give up smoking if you want to live longer, feel younger and look younger.

As far as alcohol is concerned, giving up alcohol or limiting the consumption can greatly help you feel and look more youthful.

Follow these interesting age defying tips and enjoy a more youthful you!

Feel Young as You Age – 25 Effective Anti-Aging Tips

The twenty-five anti-aging tips mentioned below are magical when it comes to slowing down your aging. Learn how to look and feel youthful as you age using these twenty-five anti-aging tips:

1. Use avocado oil: People believe avocado oil has amazing natural anti-aging properties because it can absorb into the skin tissues deeply, making it ideal for dry and mature skin. It is also loaded with sterolins, which can tremendously reduce aging spots on skin.

2. Use baby bottom butter: It is an amazing cream for women who wish to look younger. Containing lavender and olive oil for nourishing the skin gently, baby bottom butter has an interesting chamomile scent.

3. Be positive with your approach: If you remain positive about your outlook, it can work wonders on your aging skin. Negativity and worries affect you both emotionally and physically and can start to appear on your skin as you age.

4. Use a blusher: Aging turns our skin tore more ashen. A pink blusher can really help you put years off your face. Use a pink cream blush and blend it on the apples of your cheeks evenly so that it looks natural. The creamy texture is recommended because not only it gives a healthy glow to your skin but also makes it appear dewy and plump.

5. Use caffeine for skincare: Puffiness under the eyes or dark circles can be a major contributor to looking older than you really are. With the help of natural inflammatory properties of caffeine, you can reduce swelling and de-puff your eyes and can even improve circulation to get rid of dark circles. So a cream or facial moisturizer with caffeine is a must-have!

6. Collagen marshmallows: Control the effects of aging skin and try this latest trend all the way from Japan. These marshmallows are known to contain collagen peptide, which can significantly reduce aging effects on the skin.

7. Eat properly and healthy: This is the most obvious of all the tips! Healthy eating can help you stay fresh, boost your metabolism, and can even help you reduce those extra pounds that make you look older. A lot of full-fat dairy and meat can increase wrinkles. Instead, consume foods that are loaded with essential fatty acids and antioxidants like fish, veggies, and fruits. Some amazing recipes are shared in this book to help you with this.

8. The shape of your eyebrows: As we age, our eyebrows might become less defined and sparser. Thus, over-plucking your eyebrows and giving it a very sharp, thin shape can be a contributor to looking older. In fact, use a dark brow pencil and give your eyebrow a fuller, thicker shape.

9. Use eye cream: Your eyes can become wrinkly fast if you let the skin around your eyes dry. Apply some eye cream or a moisturizer near your eyes to hydrate the lines and hide the wrinkles. Gently apply the eye cream in a circular motion.

10. The choice of eye shadows: Say good bye to your metallic or wet eye shadows. The glittery or glossy particles will sit in wrinkles and lines and will make them more prominent.

11. Swap foundations with tinted moisturizer: Young skin is naturally dewy, fresh, and plump and therefore can manage heavy foundation coverage. As for you, swap it with an extra nourishing tinted moisturizer for a glowing, light look. S

12. Wear bright colors: Choose bright colors to wear, especially near your face and brighten it up. Dull colors like brown and black drain the energy and can make you look drab and old.

13. Add a little frizz to your hair: Bouncy, wavy hair gives you a very girlish touch, regardless of your age. Get rid of your straight hair and invest in some curling tongs or rollers to give them a little youthful twist.

14. Don't hesitate playing around with hair colors: Age gracefully and hide those grey hair with a color slightly lighter than your own hair color. A mix and match of dark and light shades will not only help the grey hair disappear, but will also look more natural and youthful.

15. Try using hair masks: To rehydrate overly colored or over-styled hair, treat it to a regular hot olive oil hair mask. The process is very simple, heat some oil, massage on your scalp, and cover your head and hair with a warm towel soaked in hot water. Shiny, healthy, and flowing hair will knock off age from your face.

16. Hair volume treatment: If aging has thin your hair, you can look older than you are. Curling and pulling off wavy hair can help you with that temporarily but you can go for a proper and permanent treatment. Oiling is one effective way to bring back hair volume.

17. Take care of your hands: Don't forget to moisturizer your hands with a proper hand cream on a regular basis. Hands can be the first think to show off your age. Some great moisturizer homemade recipes are shared in this book to help you with this.

18. Use jojoba oil for healthier skin: Jojoba minimizes wrinkles and fine lines and makes your skin baby soft. While jojoba oil can be a little expensive to purchase, a few drops can do wonders and thus it is worthwhile to invest in such a magical ingredient.

19. Be happy: Laughing with all your heart can also keep wrinkles and other aging effects at bay. A good laugh can help you with stress management and stay energized and refreshed.

20. Change your lipstick collection: It's time to get rid of all the dark and matte shades of lipstick that would make you look older as you age. Refill your collection with nude, natural glossy shades of pinks and browns.

21. Eat oysters to beautify your skin: While oysters are mainly known for their aphrodisiac characteristics, they are also great for your skin. Oysters contain iron

and vitamin B12, which help beat yellow or pale skin, and reduce dark circles near the eyes.

22. Perfume: Believe it or not, the way you smell can also add age to your personality. Use citrus, zesty, and fresh scents and feel youthful. A youthful smelling fragrance will actually make you appear younger.

23. Get started with a little Pilates: This form of exercise is known to strengthen body's core strength. This is done through correct breathing techniques, stretching, and balancing. Performing Pilates can take years off you, making you feel and look younger.

24. Protect your Skin: Save your skin from sun exposure as much as you can. Especially if you are aging, make sure you cover your skin with high SPF sun cream to shield your skin from the harmful rays.

25. Feel good about yourself: Sleep, rest, and enjoy and dedicate some time to yourself. Only when you are satisfied with the way you look and feel, other's will find you energetic and youthful too!

These tips can work wonders. Try them yourself!

Natural Homemade Recipes for Amazing Aging Skin

Enjoy making your own anti-aging beauty products at home! Here are some great recipes to help you pamper your skin and look younger as you age!

Honey-Avocado Moisturizer

Let's start with a moisturizer, which is an anti-aging must! This natural moisturizer made from honey and avocado will retain moisture of your skin and act as a filler for your fine lines and wrinkles. Most importantly, this blend can improve your complexion and make your skin appear smoother. Try this recipe and use it regularly to experience youthful, and dewy natural skin.

Ingredients

Honey, 1 tbsp
¼ avocado (ripe)
Fresh cream, 3 tbsp

Preparation Method

Place honey, avocado, and fresh cream in a blender or food processor and pulse to make a smooth cream mixture.

Apply a small amount of this moisturizer on your skin. Rub gently in a circular motion all over your face and leave it on for 45-60 minutes. Use warm water to rinse it off.

You will immediately feel a very soft facial skin.

Acne Spot Treatment

Acne can attack when you are aging. Aging can make acne worse and can leave blemishes on your skin. When you want to clear your skin from any and all marks, this treatment will surely help. The lemon used in this recipe will dry the blemishes while the yeast will fight the bacteria.

Ingredients

Water, 2-3 tbsp
Lemon juice (fresh), a squeeze
Brewer's years, 1 tbsp

Preparation Method

Add brewer's yeast in a mixing bowl. Add lemon and water and whisk to combine all ingredients together. Whisk for a while until it forms a thick paste.

Apply the paste only on the blemishes or acne area gently with your fingers. Leave it on for 10 minutes, covering with a bandage.

Remove the bandage and rinse it off with plain water.

Pure Basil Toner

If aging brought you acne problem, use this magical, natural toner to fight it off. Basil has been used as a main ingredient in this recipe. It behaves as a natural antiseptic, improves circulation in the skin, and helps clear bacteria that cause acne.

Ingredients

Boiling water, 1 cup
Basil leaves (dried), 3 tbsp

Preparation Method

Crush the dried basil leaves in a bowl and add to a cup of hot, boiling water.

Stir and allow the mixture to cool. When the mixture is completely cool, strain (reserving the liquid) and discard the leaves. Pour the liquid in a spray bottle and use to spray on your face.

With the help of a cotton pad, gently spread the natural basil toner around your face and neck. Before cleansing your skin, clear your skin with this toner daily.

Agave Lemon Age Spot Fighter

As mentioned earlier, your hands are the first to suffer and show off your aging. However, if you can make this scrub at home, you can fight off age spots. Exfoliate your hands get rid of the top layer of dead or damaged skin cells.

The agave in this recipe helps hydrate the skin, while the rice is used for its exfoliating properties and lemon for lightening the skin.

Ingredients

Cooked rice, ½ cup
Agave nectar, 1 tbsp
Lemon juice, 1 tbsp

Preparation Method

Add rice, agave nectar, and lemon juice in a blender and combine well.

When the mixture is prepared, apply to your dry hands and scrub gently in a circular motion. Apply gentle pressure as you scrub the back of your hands for a few minutes. Now rub this mixture on the palms of your hands to and rinse off with plain water.

Sugar-Almond Facial Scrub

Just like your hands, your face skin requires exfoliation too to get rid of the top layer of dead skin cells. Use this amazing facial scrub to lighten your complexion and make your skin look brighter and smoother.

Ingredients

Olive oil, 2 tbsp
Ground almonds, ½ cup
Brown sugar, ½ cup
White sugar, 1 cup
Fresh cream, 3 tbsp

Preparation Method.

Add all the ingredients to a mixing bowl one by one and whisk thoroughly to combine well. Apply the scrub to your dry face in a circular motion, gently using the tips of your fingers.

After a few minutes of massaging, wash off your face with warm water and then wash again with cold water. Pat dry your face with a soft towel.

Place in an airtight container or jar and store in your refrigerator for future use.

Coconut Deep Conditioner

As we all know, aging affects hair as much as it affects skin and health. Use this deep condition made of natural coconut to keep your hair shiny, hydrated, and smooth with this conditioning treatment. Use at least once a weak.

Ingredients

Coconut extract, 1 tsp
Coconut oil, 1 tbsp
Mayonnaise, ½ cu

Preparation Method

Add all ingredients to a mixing bowl and whisk to combine. Apply this paste on your scalp and cover your head with clear plastic wrap.

Leave the conditioner on for 20-30 minutes before you wash your hair and rinse it thoroughly with plain water.

Java Lip Exfoliator

Enjoy fuller and luscious lips even when you are aging and get rid of dead, dry skin from your lips. This exfoliator will instantly make your lips appear pinker and plumper.

Ingredients

Moisturizing lotion (such as Active Hydrating Body Fluid by Olay), ½ tsp
Fresh coffee grounds, ¼ tsp
Kosher salt, ¼ tsp

Preparation Method

Combine all ingredients in a bowl. Apply on your lips and outer lips area and massage gently for a few minutes.

Wipe clean with a wet and warm washcloth gently for amazing results.

Skin Texture Refiner

Refine the texture and tone of your skin with this amazing, homemade recipe. The walnuts used in this recipe are used to buff away oil, dirt, and dead skin from the face while the lactic acid present in yogurt is known for tightening pores and refining texture. Use the almond oil for moisturizing and soothing your skin for a smoother, softer feel.

Ingredients

2 whole walnuts
Yogurt, 2 tbsp
Pure almond oil, 1 tsp

Preparation Method

Crush the walnuts and combine with yogurt. Stir in almond oil and whisk together to form a paste. Use this natural exfoliant on your skin and massage for a few minutes.

Leave it on for a few minutes and then wash to clean.

Use daily for great results.

Anti-Aging Face Pack

This is an awesome face pack recipe to get rid of your wrinkles. Use twice in a week for great results. The natural ingredients used in this recipe are extremely healthy for your skin and have adverse effects on the aging, wrinkly skin.

Ingredients

Lentils, 1cup
Cream of milk, 2 tbsp
Honey, 2 tsp
Water, 2 tsp

Preparation Method

Thoroughly wash the lentils. Add them to a blender with some water and pulse to form a paste. Add honey and cream of milk to the paste and blend again to combine.

Gently apply on your skin as a face pack and leave it on for 20-25 minutes. You will feel the tightening sensation on your skin as you leave the face pack on. Wash with plain water and apply a moisturizer for glowing skin.

Natural Cracked Heel Recipe

Time to pamper your dry and cracked heels! Don't forget to take care of your feet as you age. This method can also be used to treat dry and patchy hands.

Ingredients

Olive oil (extra-virgin if possible), 1 tsp

What to do

Apply a little olive oil on your feet gently and cover with socks. Similarly, apply on your hands, cover with gloves, and leave it on overnight.

Repeat daily and expect the cracks to subside, heels and hands to be smoother in just a few days!

Moisturizing Body Cream for Aging Skin

Prepare this excellent moisturizing body cream for aging skin using essential oils of geranium, neroli, and myrrh for dry skin. The ingredients used in this recipe are great for mature, dry skin and the wheatgerm oil and vitamin E in the recipe will act as natural preservatives for a glowing skin.

Ingredients

Rosewater, ½ cup
Glycerin, 1 tbsp
Apricot kernel oil, 2 ½ tbsp
Jojoba oil, 2 tbsp
Rosehip oil, 1 tbsp
Wheatgerm oil, 1 tbsp
Avocado oil, 1 tbsp
Emulsifying wax, 2-3 tbsp
Myrrh essential oil, 4 drops
Geranium essential oil, 12 drops
Neroli essential oil, 12 drops

Preparation Method

Combine all oils (leaving essential oils aside) along with emulsifying wax in a Pyrex jug. Heat the combination using bain marie method.

In another heatproof jug, combine glycerin with rosewater and set in a microwave to heat. Once the wax has melted, stir to combine with the oils and remove from heat.

The temperature of oils and water-glycerin mixture should be almost equal. Add water-glycerin mixture to the oils in portions and whisk continuously to combine.

You can even use a hand blender at low-speed to combine all the ingredients well. Continue whisking for a few minutes until the mixture starts to solidify and cool. Add essential oils to the mixture and stir well to combine.

To store, pour in a sterilized airtight jar and store in a cool, dark place.

Apply this amazing moisturizer on your body (can also be used on the face) at least once in a day. It could give you a very oily feel at first but eventually will absorb in the skin, making you feel wonderful and soft.

Dry Skin Cleanser

Aging skin needs extra care during the winter months. Use this homemade cleanser for maturing, dry skin and feel amazing and youthful.

Ingredients

Extra virgin olive oil, 2 tbsp
Milk, ½ cup
Grapeseed oil, a few drops

Preparation Method

Combine olive oil with milk and stir to combine well. Add a few drops of grapeseed oil in the mixture and combine well.

Use this mixture to rinse your skin thoroughly. Let the oil absorb and remove excess oil patting your skin with a soft cloth. Rinse off with water.

The combination of ingredients used here provides excellent nourishment for aging skin.

Oily Skin Cleanser

Excess oil on your skin can also cause problems to aging skin. In order to prevent breakouts, use this oily skin cleanser you can easily prepare at home:

Ingredients

Raw honey, 1 tbsp
Natural oats, 1 tbsp
Ground almonds, 1 tbsp

Preparation Method

Combine honey with ground almonds and oats. Mix well to combine all ingredients. Your cleanser is now prepared.

To exfoliate and cleanse, rub the concoction on your skin gently in a circular motion. Use your fingers to focus on the T-zone more. Rinse clean with tepid water.

To store, pour the mixture in any airtight container. This cleanser can be stored for up to a week.

Note: If you have very oily skin, add a few drops of lemon to the concoction for desirable results.

Homemade Anti-Aging Mask

Fight fine lines and wrinkles the natural way with this weekly mask treatment, especially designed for maturing skin. The strawberries in this mask helps remove bacteria and bring plenty of antioxidants. On the other hand, egg whites bring protein to add nutrients and withdraw impurities from the skin.

Ingredients

Strawberries (stem removed), a handful
2 egg whites only

Preparation Method

With the help of a wooden spoon, pulverize the strawberries. Add egg whites with strawberries and whisk together with a fork to form even consistency.

Your mask is now prepared. Apply mask to freshly cleansed skin, paying special attention to areas with fine lines and wrinkles. Also, apply the mask to the neck and jaw line.

Leave it on for 5-10 minutes and then rinse with plain water. Apply moisturizer later.

Natural Anti-Aging Secrets From Around the World: Recipes from the Natives

From drinking one gallon water in a day for glowing and plump skin to brushing your hair at least 100 times, we have literally heard countless advice from our grandmothers when it comes to anti-aging tips and tricks.

Our ancestors are always ready to guide us with their experience and that is true about women from all over the world and across different cultures.

The following are some native trips from five different countries and cultures for anti aging. If you wish to go beyond the boundary to age gracefully and beautifully, these tips might be of great help to you.

China

Many Chinese teas are considered rich in anti-aging antioxidants. Green and white tea are high in a special antioxidant known as EGCG, which helps increase cell count and battle wrinkle. Here's a great anti-aging mask recipe all the way from China.

Ingredients

Green tea powder, 1 tsp – 2 tsp
Brewed white tea, ½ cup

Preparation Method

Add green tea powder to cool brewed white tea and whisk to combine. If you want thicker paste, add more green tea powder and combine.

Now apply this mask to your face, especially on wrinkly areas. Leave it on for 20-30 minutes, allow the antioxidants to fight wrinkles and plump your skin. Wash off with plain water and experience softer, smoother skin.

India

Women in India believe that consuming a hot cup of ginger tea in the morning is a great anti-aging tip. Here's a recipe that work.

Ingredients

Ginger (shredded), ½ tbsp
Honey, 1 tbsp
Hot water, 1 cup

Preparation Method

Add honey and shredded ginger in a cup of hot water and stir to combine. Drink first thing in the morning and gain maximum anti-aging benefits of natural antioxidant and anti bacterial properties this tea has to offer.

Mexico

As mentioned earlier, our hands can give the first signal of our aging. People in Mexico believe the same and that's why share this magical recipe with you.

Ingredients

Sugar, 1 tbsp
Lemon juice, 2 tbsp

Preparation Method

Whisk together lemon juice and sugar to prepare an exfoliating scrub for your hands. Apply the scrub on the top side of your hands and massage gently for a few minutes.

Wash with plan water after a few minutes for excellent results.

Polynesia

Have you heard about the noni juice? Models these days are raving about this new, natural beauty product. While the product has been around for thousands of years, the recognition it gained today has really made it popular.

Polynesians use this fruit for its natural anti-aging and moisturizing properties. So there's no secret recipe here. You just need to consume it to gain benefits of its anti-aging properties.

France

According to studies, grape seed extract supplements are beneficial for boosting antioxidants in your body. The ingredient is also known to protect the level of elastin and collagen in your skin – the essential proteins that provide your skin with firmness and elasticity.

This natural supplement is extremely popular in France. 50 mg of this natural supplement can give you similar benefits as you would get from consuming a pound of grapes.

Eating Well, Looking Younger: Super Foods for Anti-Aging

Foods, essential oils, and herbs are complex and hold a number of benefits for aging skin. Here is a list of super foods, essential oils, and herbs that work wonders in taking care of your anti-aging skin.

Foods, Herbs and Essential Oils

Foods:

1. Egg Whites: Tightening effects, vitamin E, draws out toxins
2. Apple: Ph balancing quality, reduce brown spots, smoothes skin, exfoliates
3. Honey: natural antibiotic and anti-inflammatory properties, hydrating
4. Tomato: balances pH, exfoliates, fights free radicals, protects from sun
5. Milk: lightens and exfoliates skin, rejuvenate the production of collagen
6. Carrot: builds elasticity and rejuvenates deeper skin layers
7. Yogurt: hydrates, soothes irritation, calms skin
8. Apple cider vinegar: reduces irritation, redness, and balances Ph
9. Banana: neutralizes skin acidity, nourishes, and hydrates
10. Lemon: exfoliates, removes dead skin cells
11. Oatmeal: Reduce skin irritation, attracts moisture, and exfoliates
12. Potato: Treat acne, removes excess oil, reduces swelling, relieves puffy or dark circles
13. Avocado: feeds and moisturizes skin with good fats
14. Seaweed: plums and feeds the skin, and draws out toxins
15. Pumpkin: moisturizes, soothes, remove impurities, heal skin, and revitalizes skin
16. Watermelon: protects and feeds the skin, tighten pores, clear blemishes
17. Coconut oil: prevent age spots, skin sagging, and wrinkles

Essential Oils:

1. Lavender: speed up the process of new skin cells generation, and soothes skin
2. Neroli: Regenerates damaged skin cells and improves elasticity of skin
3. Myrrh: tones skin and smoothes wrinkles
4. Carrot Seeds: has excellent toning and regenerating effects for mature skin.
5. Rose: effective for wrinkles and dry skin
6. Sandalwood: smoothes maturing skin and helps strengthen tissues

Herbs:

1. Aloe Vera: decreases redness and inflammation, draws out toxins and accelerates cell generation
2. Chamomile: reduce oiliness and helps soften
3. Elder Flowers: fade freckles, reduce wrinkles, whitens and softens skin

4. Eyebright: smoothes and soothes skin near your eyes
5. Marshmallow Root: soothes sunburns and soften skin
6. Nettle: reduces dark circles and stimulates circulation
7. Horsetail: firms, tones and helps reduce eyelid swelling
8. Lady's Mantle: has binding and toning effect on saggy, aging skin
9. Chervil: keeps skin supple and reduce wrinkles

All these ingredients are excellent, especially for aging skin. Also, they are easily available and convenient to purchase because most them are inexpensive. It is important to remember that homemade anti-aging products are free of chemical preservatives and thus you may need to make fresh batches often.

Before applying any homemade product on your face, test some on your leg or arm to see if you have any allergy or any adverse reaction from it.

Juicing the Years Off: Juicing Recipes for a Younger, Fresher You

There are claims that juicing may not only slow down aging, but can reverse the effects of aging. A number of studies prove that it is right.

The following are some popular juicing recipes to help you enjoy and reverse the signs of aging:

Turnip Fennel Juice

Prepare this great juice loaded with manganese and vitamin C.

Ingredients

¼ fennel bulb
1 medium-sized apple
3 medium-sized carrots (peeled)
½ turnip

Preparation Method

Blend all the ingredients together in a food processor or blender and enjoy.

Parsley Explosion

Parsley juice is extremely potent and full of energy. It is filled with chlorophyll that oxygenates blood and refresh your skin.

Ingredients

1 celery
1 medium-sized apple
2 medium-sized carrots (peeled)
Parsley, 1 large bunch

Preparation Method

Juice together all the ingredients, keeping apple to juice last.

Shake, drink and enjoy!

Parsnip Orange Juice

Parsnips are naturally sweet and are an excellent source of manganese, folate, and vitamin C.

Ingredients

1 medium-sized apple
1 celery stalk
½ orange
2 medium-sized carrots
3 parsnips

Preparation Method

Blend all the ingredients together in a high speed blender and enjoy the sweet, natural taste of this healthy juice.

Eggplant and Carrot Blend

Darker vegetables are considered richer in antioxidants. Eggplant is an excellent ingredient to add to this juicing recipe for desirable results.

Ingredients

1 celery stalk
2 medium-sized carrots
2 medium-sized apples
1 eggplant

Preparation Method

Juice the entire eggplant, along with its skin and seeds, and blend with the remaining ingredients and relish.

Swiss Chard Meets Kale Juice

Loaded with minerals and vitamins, you just can't ignore this recipe made up Swiss Chard.

Ingredients

2 medium-sized apples
2 celery stalks
2 medium-sized carrots
Kale (1 cup)
Swiss Chard, 2 cups

Preparation Method

Juice all the green ingredients first. Add the remaining ingredients to the blender and prepare a rich and healthy juice.

Red Pepper Beauty Blend

Red peppers used in this recipe can improve your skin due to the level of carotenoids present in them.

Ingredients

1 broccoli spear
1 medium-sized apple
2 medium-sized carrots
2 red peppers

Ingredients

Juice all the ingredients together and drink this beauty blend for great complexion and flawless skin.

Orange Blush

Delicious and fruity – this drink is surely a great way to kickstart your day!

Ingredients

6 large carrots (peeled)
2 medium-sized apples
1 pineapple

Preparation Method

Blend all the fruits in a high speed blender and refresh yourself with a glass of this fruity blend.

Everyday Cleanser

Enjoy a high nutrient, flavorful drink and take 10 years off your face and skin.

Ingredients

Turmeric or ginger (a small piece)
1 medium-sized cucumber
4 celery stalks
2 medium-sized carrots (peeled)
1 medium-sized apple
kale, 4-6 leaves

Preparation Method

Combine all ingredients in a juicer or fruit processor until smooth. Pour in your favorite glass and relish for a daily body cleanser.

Wrinkle 'Beeter'

Rich in nutrients and exotic flavors, this healthy blend is surely going to do great benefits to your skin.

Ingredients

½ lemon
1 medium-sized apple
2-4 carrots
Kale, 4-6 leaves
Red beet with stalks, one small

Preparation Method

Add all ingredients in a blender and pulse until it forms juice. Enjoy the flavorful blend in your favorite glass.

Immortality Juice

A blend of healthy fruits and vegetables definitely makes this juice a must-have for anti-aging purpose.

Ingredients

Garlic, 1 clove
4 celery stalks
4 medium-sized carrots
1 green apple
Kale, 2-4 leaves
Parsley, a bunch
2 large-sized tomatoes

Preparation Method

Combine all the ingredients in a bowl before you put them to the blender. Pulse it at high to juice instantly. Serve yourself with a healthy blend immediately.

Have you ever thought your eating habits and choice of ingredients can also help you age as gracefully as you like? We have some amazing anti-aging recipes to share with you in the next chapter.

Recipes to Relish

So here we have some of the most interesting, anti-aging recipes you can enjoy. Prepare your favorite one now and enjoy delicious, healthy food as you age!

Buffalo Mozzarella Anchovies, Capers and Olives on Sourdough

Ingredients

Sourdough bread, 4 slices
Anchovy fillets (marinated), 16
Buffalo mozzarella (chunks), 5 oz
8 olives (green, chopped)
Extra-virgin olive oil, 3 tbsp
Red wine vinegar, 2 tbsp

Preparation Method

1. First, toast sourdough slices, until brown. Divide the mozzarella chunks between 4 slices of bread and place four anchovy fillets over the mozzarella on each slice.
2. In a small bowl, combine olive oil, olives, and capers and drizzle the seasoning over the mozzarella.
3. Serve immediately and relish.

Sweet and Sour Cabbage with Salmon

Ingredients

Olive oil, 2 tbsp
1 head small-sized red cabbage (cored and sliced thinly)
1 medium-sized sweet onion (sliced thinly)
Pepper, to taste
Salt, to taste
Balsamic vinegar, 2 tbsp
Dry red wine, ½ cup
Blackberries, ½ pint
Centre-cut salmon fillets (skinless), 4 pieces
Parsley (chopped), for topping

Preparation Method

1. Heat oil in a deep skillet over med-high flame. Add onion and sauté until tender, stirring constantly.
2. Add cabbage to the skillet and sprinkle salt and black pepper and cook until it starts to wilt, for around 3-4 minutes, stirring constantly. Add vinegar and wine and allow boiling.
3. Cover with lid and let it simmer until tender over low-med heat, for around 20 minutes. Remove from stove, add blackberries to the skillet, and set aside.
4. Set he broiler to preheat and prepare a jelly-roll pan with foil. Place fish fillets over the pan and season with salt and pepper.
5. Broil fillets for 7-8 minutes. Pour cabbage mixture equally in serving plates, place salmon over it, and top with parsley for best flavors.
6. Enjoy!

Grilled Mackerel with Fennel and Pink Grapefruit Salad

Ingredients

Mackerel fish, 4 fillets
½ fennel bulb (thinly sliced)
1 large-sized pink grapefruit, (segmented and reserve juices)
Olive oil, 2 tbsp + more
Dill (remove sprigs), 1 small bunch
Salt, to taste
Black pepper, to taste

Preparation Method

1. Set the grill to high heat. Prepare fish fillets, brushing it with olive oil and seasoning it with salt and pepper.
2. Set to grill until skin is translucent, for about 6-8 minutes. Combine oil and grapefruit juice in a bowl.
3. Stir through grapefruit and fennel with the dill. Season and place over fish fillets.
4. Your fish is now prepared. Place on a serving platter and accompany with steamed potatoes to complete the meal.

Linguine with Turkey-Carrot Ragu

Ingredients

Olive oil, 1 tbsp
celery (chopped), 2 stalks
1 large-sized leek, (only light green and white parts, well rinsed and sliced)
Lean ground turkey, 1 lb
Garlic (minced), 2 cloves
Salt, to taste
Pepper, to taste
Ground cinnamon, 1 tsp
Canned tomatoes (diced, no added salt), 2 cans
Whole wheat linguine, 8 oz
Carrots, 1 lb
Fresh parsley (chopped), 1 tbsp

Preparation Method

1. Add water and some salt to 5-quart pot and set to boil over high heat.
2. In a large skillet, heat oil over med-high flame. Add garlic, celery, leek, pepper, and salt in the skillet and cook until tender, for around 5 minutes, stirring constantly.
3. Next, add turkey to the skillet and cook for another 4-5 minutes, breaking it into small pieces, and stirring constantly. Stir in tomatoes and cinnamon, heat until the mixture boils, and then allow simmering over low heat for at least 10-15 minutes.
4. Meanwhile, using a veggie peeler, shave carrots like thin ribbons.
5. Add linguine to boiling, salted water and cook according to package directions.1 minute before the pasta is done, add carrots and cook along with carrots.
6. Drain well and return to the pot. Add more pepper and salt along with turkey ragu you have prepared, and stir gently to combine well.
7. Top with parsley and your dish is ready to be served.

Broad Bean Noodles with Thai Beef Salad

Ingredients

Toasted peanuts (chopped), 4 tbsp
Fresh coriander (chopped), 4 tbsp
Sirloin steak, 3 steaks about 1-inch thick
Ready-cooked noodles, 10 oz.
4 spring onions (thinly sliced)
Green beans (refreshed, blanched, and trimmed), 7oz.
3 medium-sized carrots
1 medium-sized cucumber

Ingredients for Dressing

Juice of 1 lime
Sweet chili, 1 tbsp
Rice vinegar, 2 tbsp
Thai fish sauce, 2 tbsp
Agave syrup, 1 tbsp

Preparation Method

1. To prepare the dressing, combine all the ingredients well and set aside.
2. To prepare the salad, first peel off the cucumber and carrots. Now peel the flesh, dragging it all the way down, and stop when you reach the seeds. Repeat with carrots.
3. Toss the carrot and cucumber shavings with green beans, and spring onions. Add ½ of the dressing and toss to combine.
4. Heat oil in a frying pan over low-med heat and fry noodles for 1-2 minutes. When done, allow to cool and combine with the salad mix.
5. Heat the pan again, grease with oil. Lightly oil the steak and season with salt and pepper. Cook steak, 3-4 minutes or longer, on the pan.
6. To serve, cut steaks into strip and combine with the salad. Stir in peanuts and coriander and toss again. Serve immediately!

California Breakfast Wrap

Ingredients

4 large-sized eggs (with yolk)
2 large-sized eggs (only white)
4 large whole wheat tortillas
Baby spinach, 6 cups
Goat cheese, 4 tbsp
Salt, to taste
Black pepper, to taste
Canola oil, 1 tsp
1 avocado (chopped)
1 medium-sized tomato (finely chopped)
Fresh dill leaves (chopped), 1 tbsp

Preparation Method

1. Beat egg whites, eggs, a pinch of salt and pepper in a bowl.
2. Place tortillas on microwavable plate and cover with slightly damp paper tower. Set to heat in a microwave for 30 seconds.
3. When tortillas are warm, add 1 tbsp of goat cheese over each tortilla, and spread evenly. Top with lots of spinach.
4. Heat oil in a large skillet over low-med heat. Add the egg mixture and cook for a few minutes, stirring constantly. Remove from heat, season with more salt, and fold in avocado and tomato.
5. Divide egg into four equal portions and place over tortillas. Garnish with dill and wrap it up before serving.

Scallop Ceviche and Salmon with Lime and Avocado Recipe

Ingredients

Juice of 3 lemons
Juice of 1 orange
Juice of 3 limes
Caster sugar, 1 tbsp
1 ½ red chili (finely sliced)
½ red onion (diced)
4 kind scallops (sliced, remove roe)
1 avocado (slice into small chunks)
Salmon fillets (finely sliced and skinless), 10oz.
Coriander (chopped), a handful
Cherry tomatoes (quartered), 5 oz
Sea salt, to taste
Black pepper, to taste

Preparation Method

1. Combine lemon, lime, and orange juices in a bowl. Stir in some salt, sugar, chili, and onion and combine. Let it sit for 60 minutes, taste and adjust seasoning and sweetness, if required.
2. Place the fillets and scallops in the citrus dressing and toss to combine. Cover with plastic wrap and set to refrigerate for 1 hour, until the scallops and fish appear opaque.
3. Stir tomatoes, avocado, and coriander in the seafood-vegetable mixture. With the help of a slotted spoon, pull fish out from the juice and serve. Put green salad and crusty bread on the side and serve!

Whole-Grain Blueberry Muffins

Ingredients

Whole wheat flour, 1 cup
Oats (old-fashioned, uncooked), 1 cup
Baking powder, 2 tsp
All-purpose flour, ½ cup
Baking soda, ½ tsp
Salt, ½ tsp
Brown sugar, ¼ cup + 1 tbsp
Buttermilk (low-fat), 1 cup
Orange juice (fresh), ¼ cup
1 large egg
Vanilla extract, 1 tsp
Blueberries, 2 cup
Almonds (chopped), ¼ cup

Preparation Method

1. Set the oven to preheat 400°F. Prepare muffin pan (12-cup) with liners.
2. Place oats in a food processor and pulse to grind. In a mixing bowl, whisk flours, oats, baking soda, baking powder, sugar (¼ cup), and salt. In another bowl, whisk buttermilk, vanilla, egg, oil, and juice. Stir wet mixture into dry mixture until it makes a thick batter.
3. Stir in blueberries and mix again. Stir in remaining sugar and nuts.
4. Spoon the mixture into the muffins pan, sprinkling sugar and almond on top. Set to bake until done, for around 22 minutes.
5. Remove and place it on a wire rack and allow to cool for 5-10 minutes.
6. Remove from pan and enjoy delicious blueberry muffins.

Flounder with Tomatoes and Corn

Ingredients

Fresh kernel corn, 2 cups
Tomatoes (sundried, chopped), 1 cup
Salt, to taste
Black pepper, to taste
Lemon peel (freshly grated), 1 tsp
Flounder fillets (skinless), 4 fillets
Fresh thyme, 4 sprigs
1 small-sized leek (only white part, slice into matchstick size), rinse well
Dry white wine, 8 tsp
Spinach, 8 oz.
Extra virgin olive oil, 2 tsp

Preparation Method

1. Set the oven to preheat at 450°F.
2. In a large mixing bowl, combine, tomatoes, peel, corn, and season with some pepper and salt.
3. Prepare a large baking sheet, covering it with foil or parchment paper. Arrange vegetables (¼ portions) on a side of the baking sheet. Fold 1 fillet into thirds and adjust it on top. Cover with leek (¼ portions), 2 tsp wine, 1 thyme sprig, some salt, and ½ tsp oil.
4. Fold the other side of the foil or parchment paper to cover the fish fillet. Fold the other corner and make a packet. Repeat the process to make 4 packs for 4 fillets and set to bake for 15 minutes.
5. In a glass tray or bowl, place spinach and cover with damp paper towel. Set to microwave for 2-3 minutes. Season with salt and pepper and toss to combine.
6. When you are done baking, open packets carefully, keeping your face away to avoid direct contact with steam.
7. Place opened-packets on a serving platter and side with warm spinach.

Chicken Bake with Roasted Broccoli

Ingredients

Pearl barley, 1 cup
Olive oil, 2 tbsp
Chicken broth (low sodium), 3 cups
Chicken breast halves (boneless, skinless, cut into small 1-inch pieces)
1 large-sized carrot (chopped)
Fresh thyme leaves (chopped), 2 tsp
Water, ¼ cup
Garlic (chopped), 2 cloves
1 small-sized onion (chopped)
Mushrooms (thinly sliced), 8 oz.
Broccoli florets (small), 6 cups
Salt, to taste
Black pepper, to taste

Preparation Method

1. Set the oven to preheat at 400°F.
2. In a mixing bowl, combine chicken broth and barley. Use a plastic wrap to cover it up. Set in a microwave and heat on high for 22-25 minutes, stirring once, until the liquid is completely gone.
3. Meanwhile, heat oil in a large skillet over med-high flame. Add chicken, stir, and season with pepper and salt. Stir and cook chicken for 4-5 minutes. When done, use a slotted spoon to remove chicken from the skillet and place it in a bowl.
4. Add onion, carrot, and thyme to skillet, stir, and cook for 2-3 minutes. Add garlic, stir, then add water and mushrooms. Cook for 2 minutes, stirring occasionally, and remove from heat when done.
5. Stir in barley and chicken mixture you heated and transfer all the content in the skillet to a prepared baking dish (3 quart).
6. In a bowl, toss broccoli with some olive oil and a pinch of salt and arrange the vegetable on top of the chicken mixture. Set to bake until broccoli is cooked and tender, for 22-25 minutes.
7. Serve hot and enjoy!

Sticky Chicken Wings with Lime and Lemongrass

Ingredients

Chicken wings (free-range preferable), 16 wings
Sunflower oil, ¼ cup
4 lemongrass stalks (minced)
Lime leaves (dried), 10 leaves
Thai sweet chili sauce, ¼ cup
Lime wedges, to serve

Preparation Method

1. In a large mixing bowl, add all ingredients and combine thoroughly. Cover with plastic wrap or cling film and set to refrigerate for 2 hours to overnight.
2. Set the oven to preheat at 400°F.
3. Prepare a large roasting tin and line it with greased foil. Place chicken on the foil and pour the marinade on top. Set to roast until chicken is golden for around 40 minutes. Turn chicken once halfway through roasting.
4. When done, remove from oven and serve on a platter with lime wedges on the side.

White Tea Choco Pots with Pistachio Toffee

Ingredients

Single cream, ½ cup
White tea (dunked in hot water), 3 teabags
Dark chocolate (chopped), 1 cup
Agave syrup, 6 tbsp
Roasted pistachios (chopped), 4 tbsp
1 free-range egg
Salt, a pinch

Preparation Method

1. Add cream to white tea and heat gently. Allow to cook for a few minutes until the mixture starts to steam. Remove from stove and set aside.
2. To prepare the choco pots, whizz 1 tablespoon agave syrup, chocolate and a pinch of salt in a high-power blender. Add the tea-cream mixture to the blender and pulse again to combine. Add egg in the end and whizz.
3. Divide the mixture into 8 cups, glasses or ramekins and set to refrigerate for 3-4 hours before serving.
4. Meanwhile, prepare the topping. Set a frying pan over low-med heat and heat agave syrup. Let the bubble form and cook for 2 minutes. Add pistachios, combine and remove from heat. Pour the mixture on a parchment-prepared baking sheet. Allow to cool and then break into small pieces.
5. When the chocolate pots are ready to be serves, place some pistachio toffee on the top and relish.

Goat Cheese, Walnuts and Stir-Fried Greens

Ingredients

Curly kale, ½ cup
1 cabbage (pointed)
Broccoli (tender stem), ¾ cup
Sunflower oil, 2 tbsp
Garlic (chopped), 2 cloves
Toasted walnuts, ¼ cup
Goat cheese (soft), ¾ cup
Balsamic glaze, 2-3 tbsp

Preparation Method

1. Fill a large pot with water and season with salt. Place over high heat and bring it to boil. Chop all the green vegetables and blanch for 2-3 minutes. Drain and refresh in cold water. When done, pat dry using kitchen paper.
2. Heat oil in a wok. Sauté garlic and add greens. Stir fry the veggies for a few minutes. Sprinkle a little pepper and salt. Divide and place it equally on 4 plates. Top with chopped walnuts and crumbled goat cheese.
3. Before serving, flavor with some balsamic glaze on the top and enjoy!

Enjoying Aging!

Aging is a fact of life and it comes with its own perks and drawbacks. While you cannot avoid aging, controlling the affects are pretty much in your own hand.

If you take a proactive approach, you can control signs of aging to a great extent and can age as gracefully and beautifully as you like.

This book shares all the information that will help you in this regard. Aging is a phase of life that should be enjoyed. If you take care of yourself, your skin, and especially your diet, you can not only slow down aging, but can even reverse it.

So what are you waiting for? Use the information shared in this book to your best interest and start 'Aging Gracefully' now!

Good luck!